List of Authentics Mediterranean Recipes

Living and Eating Well Every Day

Sasha Merianelli

Table of Contents

Simple Green Salad

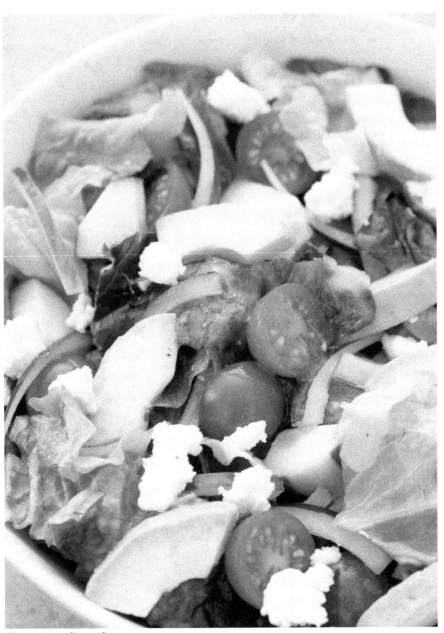

Preparation time:

5 minutes Cooking time: 5 minutes Servings: 4

Ingredients:

- ¼ cup extra-virgin olive oil
- 1 tablespoon fresh lemon juice
- ¼ teaspoon salt
- ¼ teaspoon freshly ground black pepper 6 cups loosely packed mixed greens
- ½ small red onion, thinly sliced
- 1 small cucumber, peeled and thinly sliced
- ¼ cup shredded Parmesan cheese

Directions:

1. Mix the oil, lemon juice, salt, plus pepper in a small bowl. Store the dressing in 4 condiment cups. Mix the mixed greens, onion, and cucumber in a large bowl. Divide salad into 4 medium storage containers. Top each with 1 tablespoon of Parmesan cheese. To serve, toss the dressing and salad.

Nutrition: Calories: 162g Fat: 15g Carbohydrates: 6g Fiber: 2g

Protein: 3g Sodium: 290mg

Kale-Poppy Seed Salad

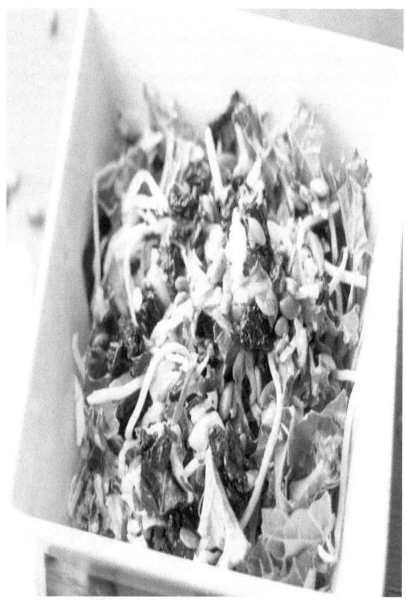

Preparation time:

10 minutes Cooking time: 5 minutes Servings: 6

Ingredients:

- ½ cup nonfat plain Greek yogurt 2 tablespoons apple cider vinegar
- ½ tablespoon extra-virgin olive oil
- 1 teaspoon poppy seeds 1 teaspoon sugar
- 4 cups firmly packed finely chopped kale
- 2 cups broccoli slaw
- 2 cups thinly sliced Brussels sprouts 6 tablespoons dried cranberries
- 6 tablespoons hulled pumpkin seeds

Directions:

1. Mix the yogurt, vinegar, oil, poppy seeds, sugar in a small bowl. Store the dressing in 6 condiment cups.

2. In a large bowl, mix the kale, broccoli slaw, and Brussels sprout. Divide the greens into 6 large storage containers and top each salad with cranberries and pumpkin seeds. To serve, toss the greens with the poppy seed dressing to coat.

Nutrition: Calories: 129g Fat: 6g

Carbohydrates: 13g Fiber: 3g

Protein: 8g

Sodium: 26mg

Edamame Salad with Corn and Cranberries

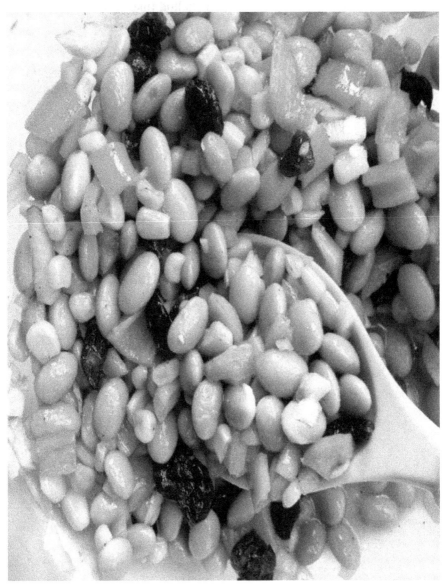

Preparation time:

15 minutes Cooking time: 0 minutes Servings: 4

Ingredients:

- 11/4 cups shelled edamame 3/4 cup corn kernels
- red or orange bell pepper, chopped
- 1/4 cup dried cranberries 1 shallot, finely diced
- tablespoons red wine vinegar
- 1 tablespoon olive oil
- 1 teaspoon agave nectar
- 1 teaspoon no-salt-added prepared mustard Freshly ground black pepper, to taste

Directions:

1. Place the edamame, corn, bell pepper, cranberries, and shallot in a mixing bowl and stir to combine. Mix the vinegar, oil, agave nectar, and mustard into a small mixing bowl.

2. Pour the dressing over the salad. Flavor with freshly ground black pepper, to taste. Serve.

Nutrition: Calories: 149

Fat: 5 g

Protein: 5 g

Sodium: 5 mg

Fiber: 3 g

Carbohydrates: 22 g

Sugar: 10 g

Warm Asian Slaw

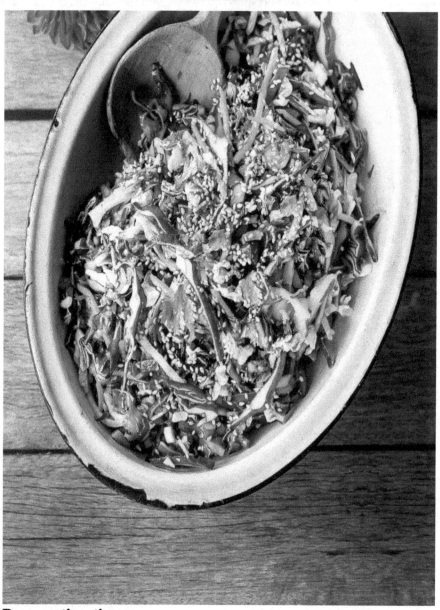

Preparation time:

15 minutes Cooking time: 3 minutes Servings: 4

Ingredients:

- tablespoon sesame oil 1 tablespoon peanut oil 2 sliced scallions
- cloves garlic, minced
- tablespoon minced fresh ginger 1 medium bok choy, chopped
- medium carrots, shredded
- 1 tablespoon unflavored rice vinegar 1/2 teaspoon sugar
- 1/2 teaspoon ground white pepper
- 1/2 tablespoon toasted sesame seeds (optional)

Directions:

1. Heat both oils in a skillet over medium. Add scallions, garlic, and ginger and cook, stirring, for 1 minute. Add bok choy and carrots and sauté for 2 minutes. Remove from heat.

2. Place contents in a bowl. Stir in vinegar, sugar, and pepper. Garnish with sesame seeds, if desired. Serve immediately.

Nutrition: Calories: 112

Fat: 7 g

Protein: 3 g

Sodium: 72 mg

Fiber: 3 g

Carbohydrates: 9 g

Sugar: 4 g

Tangy Three-Bean Salad with Barley

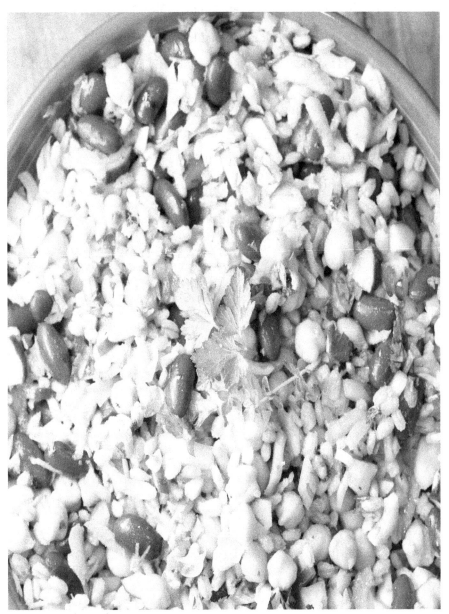

Preparation time:

15 minutes Cooking time: 30 minutes Servings: 8

Ingredients:

- cup uncooked pearled barley 21/4 cups water
- cups of green beans, slice into 2-inch pieces
- 1 (15-ounce) can no-salt-added kidney beans
- 1 (15-ounce) can no-salt-added garbanzo beans 1 medium red bell pepper, diced
- small onion, finely chopped
- tablespoons chopped fresh cilantro or parsley 1/3 cup canola oil
- 1/3 cup apple cider vinegar 1/3 cup pure maple syrup
- Freshly ground black pepper, to taste

Directions:

1. Measure the barley and water into a saucepan and boil over high heat. Once boiling, adjust heat to low, cover, and simmer until water is absorbed, 25–30 minutes. Remove pan from heat, then drain and rinse well.

2. Put the green beans in a bowl, then put the drained canned beans, bell pepper, onion, barley, and chopped cilantro or parsley. Stir well.

3. Mix the oil, vinegar, plus maple syrup in a small mixing bowl. Put on the salad and toss to coat. Flavor with ground black pepper, then serve.

Nutrition: Calories: 367

Fat: 11 g

Protein: 11 g

Sodium: 10 mg

Fiber: 11 g

Carbohydrates: 57 g

Wedge Salad with Creamy Blue Cheese Dressing

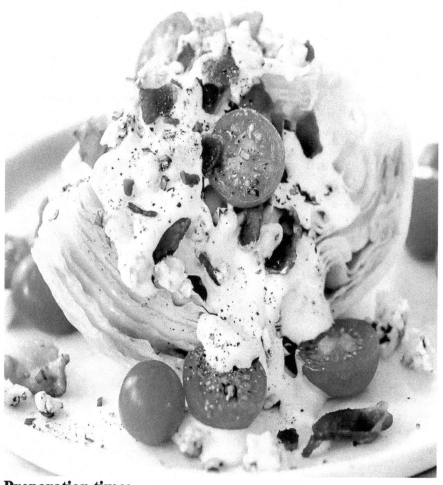

Preparation time:

15 minutes Cooking time: 0 minutes Servings: 4

Ingredients:

- cup nonfat plain Greek yogurt Juice of ½ large lemon
- ¼ teaspoon freshly ground black pepper
- ¼ teaspoon salt
- 1/3 cup crumbled blue cheese
- heads romaine lettuce, stem end trimmed, halved lengthwise 1 cup grape tomatoes, halved
- ½ cup slivered almonds

Directions:

1. Mix the yogurt, lemon juice, pepper, salt, and cheese in a small bowl. Store the dressing in 4 condiment cups. Divide the lettuce halves and tomatoes among 4 large storage containers. Store the almonds separately.

2. To serve, arrange a half-head of romaine on a plate and top with the tomatoes. Sprinkle with 2 tablespoons of almonds and drizzle with the dressing.

Nutrition: Calories: 216g Fat: 11g

Carbohydrates: 20g

Fiber: 9g Protein: 16g Sodium: 329mg

Southwestern Bean Salad with Creamy Avocado Dressing

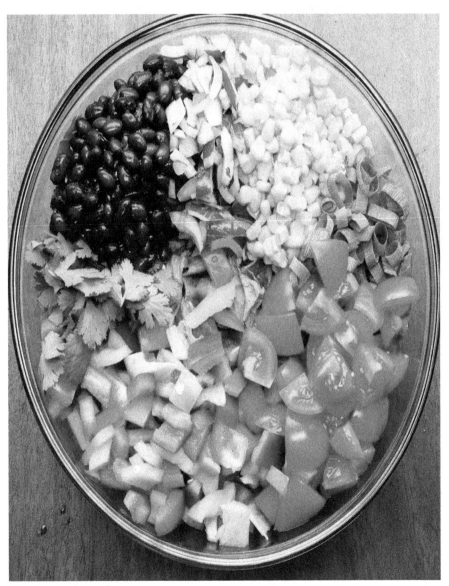

Preparation time:

15 minutes Cooking time: 0 minutes Servings: 4

Ingredients:

- 1 head romaine lettuce, chopped
- can no-salt-added black beans, drained 2 cups fresh corn kernels
- cups grape tomatoes, halved
- small avocados, halved and pitted 1 cup chopped fresh cilantro 1 cup nonfat plain Greek yogurt 8 scallions, chopped
- garlic cloves, quartered zest, and juice of 1 large lime
- ½ teaspoon sugar

Directions:

1. Mix the lettuce, beans, corn, and tomatoes in a large bowl. Toss you well combined. Divide the salad into 4 large storage containers. Put the avocado flesh into your blender or food processor.

2. Add the yogurt, scallions, garlic, lime zest and juice, and sugar. Blend until well combined. Divide the dressing into 4 condiment cups. To serve, toss the salad and the dressing.

Nutrition: Calories: 349g Fat: 11g

Carbohydrates: 53g Fiber: 16g

Protein: 19g Sodium: 77mg

Cobb Pasta Salad

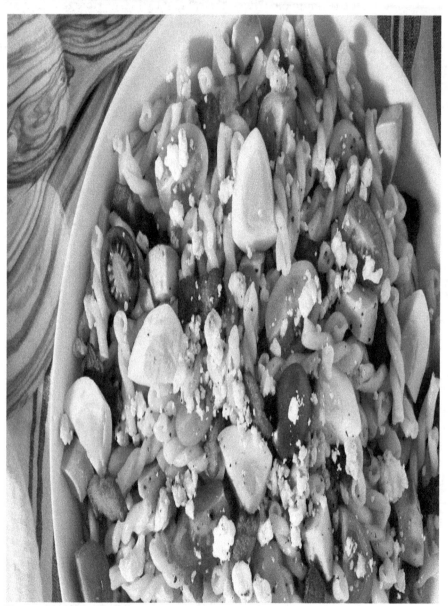

Preparation time:

15 minutes Cooking time: 10 minutes Servings: 6

Ingredients:

- 1-pound whole wheat rotini pasta
- 2 cups cooked chicken breast, chopped
- 8 low-sodium turkey bacon slices, cooked and chopped 4 scallions, sliced
- 1½ cups cherry tomatoes halved
- ¼ teaspoon freshly ground black pepper
- 4 hard-boiled eggs, peeled and coarsely chopped 1/3 cup crumbled blue cheese
- 1 cup frozen avocado cubes
- ¾ cup Greek Yogurt Dill Dressing

Directions:

1. Cook the pasta until al dente as stated to package directions. Rinse under cold water, then drain. Mix the pasta, chicken, bacon, scallions, tomatoes, pepper in a large bowl. Toss until well combined.

2. Add the eggs and blue cheese and fold until mixed well. Divide the salad into 6 storage containers. Divide the avocado into 6 small storage containers. Make the dressing as directed and store in 6 condiment cups.

3. The night before you're planning on having a salad, add the portion off the avocado to the salad so they will be soft by mealtime the next day. Serve drizzled with the dressing.

Nutrition: Calories: 550g Fat: 18g

Carbohydrates: 62g

Fiber: 9.5g Protein: 40g Sodium: 619mg

Mediterranean Pop Corn Bites

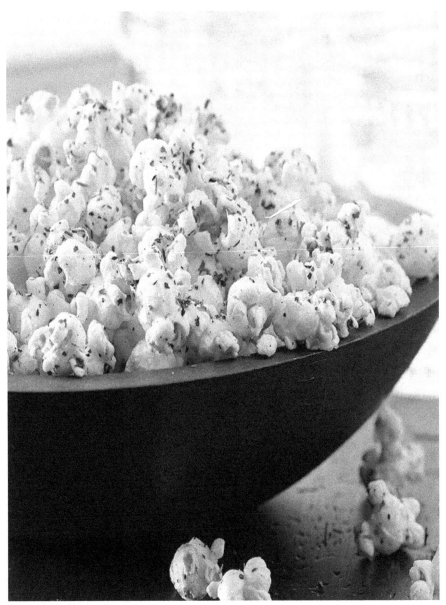

Preparation time:

5 minutes + 20 minutes chill time Cooking Time: 2-3 minutes Servings: 4

Ingredients:

- 3 cups Medjool dates, chopped 12 ounces brewed coffee
- 1 cup pecan, chopped
- ½ cup coconut, shredded
- ½ cup of cocoa powder

Directions:

1. Soak dates in warm coffee for 5 minutes. Remove dates from coffee and mash them, making a fine smooth mixture. Stir in remaining ingredients (except cocoa powder) and form small balls out of the mixture. Coat with cocoa powder, serve and enjoy!

Nutrition: Calories: 265 Fat: 12g

Carbohydrates: 43g Protein 3g

Sodium: 75 mg

Hearty Buttery Walnuts

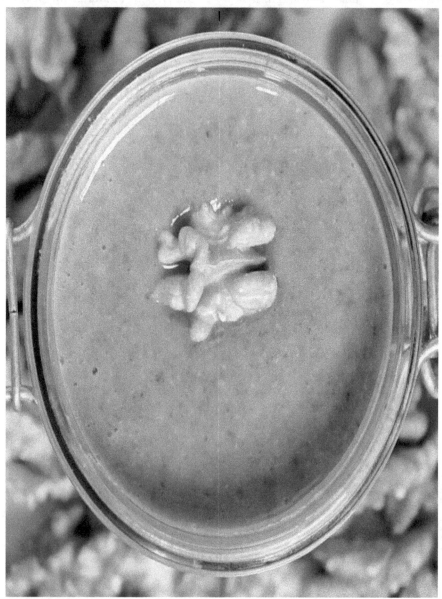

Preparation time:

10 minutes Cooking Time: 0 minutes Servings: 4

Ingredients:

- 4 walnut halves
- ½ tablespoon almond butter

Directions:

1. Spread butter over two walnut halves. Top with other halves. Serve and enjoy!

Nutrition: Calories: 90 Fat: 10g

Carbohydrates: 0g Protein: 1g Sodium: 1 mg

Refreshing Watermelon Sorbet

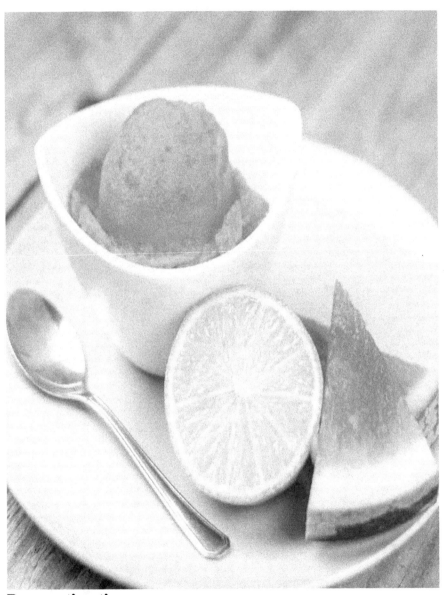

Preparation time:

20 minutes + 20 hours chill time Cooking Time: 0 minutes

Servings: 4

Ingredients:

- cups watermelon, seedless and chunked
- ¼ cup of coconut sugar 2 tablespoons lime juice

Directions:

1. Add the listed fixing to a blender and puree. Freeze the mix for about 4- 6 hours until you have gelatin-like consistency.

2. Puree the mix once again in batches and return to the container. Chill overnight. Allow the sorbet to stand for 5 minutes before serving and enjoy!

Nutrition: Calories: 91 Fat: 0g

Carbohydrates: 25g Protein: 1g Sodium: 0mg

Garlic Cottage Cheese Crispy

Preparation time:

5 minutes Cooking Time: 2 minutes Servings: 4

Ingredients:

- 1 cup cottage cheese
- ½ teaspoon Garlic powder Pinch of pepper
- Pinch of onion powder

Directions:

1. Take a bowl and mix in cheese and spices. Scoop half a teaspoon of the cheese mix and place it in the pan. Cook in a skillet over medium heat within 1 minute per side. Repeat until done.

Nutrition: Calories: 70 Fat: 6g

Carbohydrates: 1g Protein: 6g Sodium: 195 mg

Lemon Fat Bombs

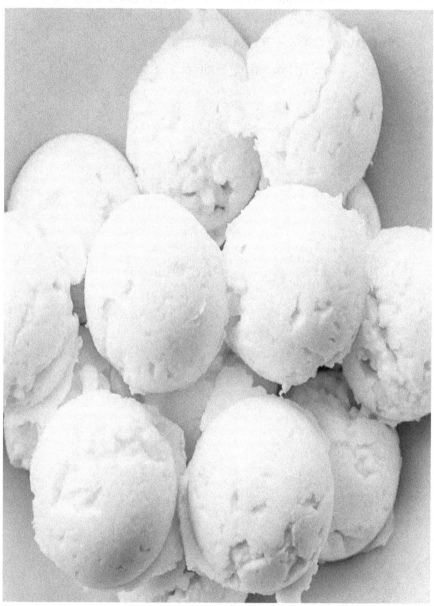

Preparation time:

10 minutes Cooking Time: 0 minutes Servings: 3

Ingredients:

- 1 whole lemon
- 4 ounces cream cheese 2 ounces butter
- 2 teaspoons natural sweetener

Directions:

2. Take a fine grater and zest your lemon. Squeeze lemon juice into a bowl alongside the zest. Add butter, cream cheese to a bowl, and add zest, salt, sweetener, and juice.

3. Stir well using a hand mixer until smooth. Spoon mix into molds and freeze for 2 hours. Serve and enjoy!

Nutrition: Calories: 404 Carbs: 4g Fiber: 1g Protein: 4g Fat: 43g Sodium: 19 mg

Chocolate Coconut Bombs

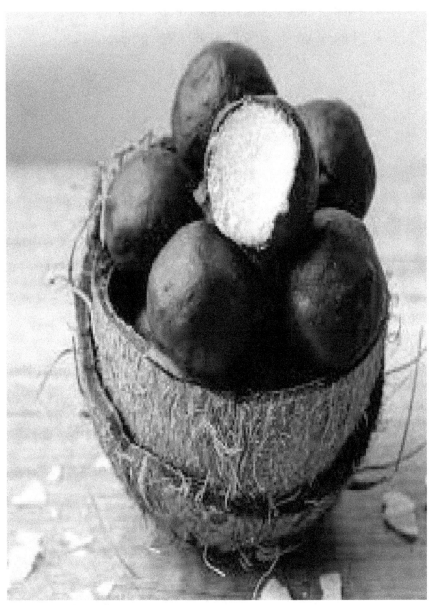

Preparation time:

20 minutes Cooking Time: 0 minutes Servings: 12

Ingredients:

- ½ cup dark cocoa powder
- ½tablespoon vanilla extract 5 drops stevia
- 1 cup coconut oil, solid 1tablespoon peppermint extract

Directions:

1. Take a high-speed food processor and add all the ingredients. Blend until combined. Take a teaspoon and drop a spoonful onto parchment paper. Refrigerate until solidified and keep refrigerated.

Nutrition: Calories: 126 Carbs: 0g Fiber: 0g Protein: 0g Fat: 14g Sodium: 30 mg

Espresso Fat Bombs

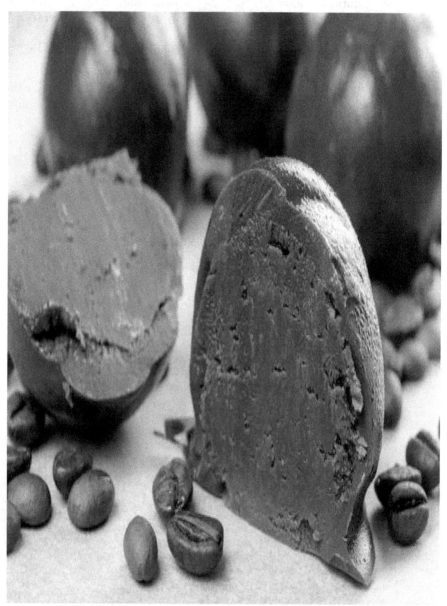

Preparation time:

20 minutes Cooking Time: 0 minutes Servings: 24

Ingredients:

- 5 tablespoons butter, tender 3 ounces cream cheese, soft 2 ounces espresso
- 4 tablespoons coconut oil
- 2 tablespoons coconut whipping cream 2 tablespoons stevia

Directions:

2. Prepare your double boiler and melt all ingredients (except stevia) for 3-4 minutes and mix. Add sweetener and mix using a hand mixer.

3. Spoon mixture into silicone muffin molds and freeze for 4 hours. Remove fat bombs and serve!

Nutrition: Carbs: 1.3g Fiber: 0.2g Protein: 0.3g Fat: 7g Sodium: 50 mg

Crispy Coconut Bombs

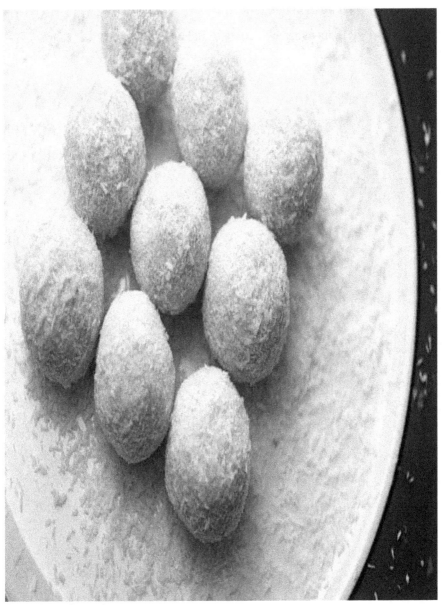

Preparation time:

10 minutes Cooking Time: 0 minutes Servings: 6

Ingredients:

- 14 ½ ounces coconut milk
- ¾ cup of coconut oil
- cup unsweetened coconut flakes 20 drops stevia

Directions:

1. Microwave your coconut oil for 20 seconds in the microwave. Mix in coconut milk and stevia in the hot oil. Stir in coconut flakes and pour the mixture into molds. Let it chill for 60 minutes in the fridge. Serve and enjoy!

Nutrition: Carbs: 2g Fiber: 0.5g Protein: 1g Fat: 13g Calories: 123 Carbs: 1g Sodium: 0mg

Pumpkin Pie Fat Bombs

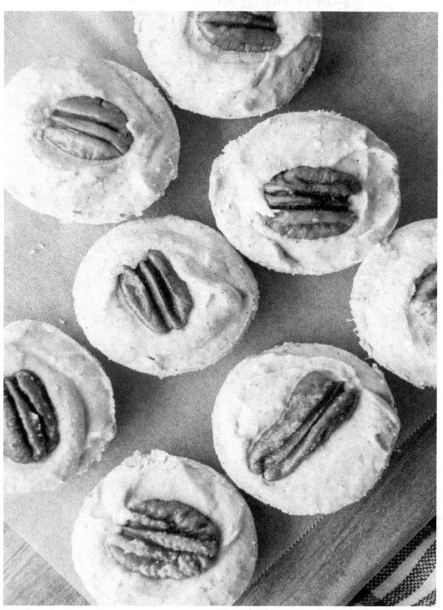

Preparation time:

35 minutes Cooking Time: 5 minutes Servings: 12

Ingredients:

- tablespoons coconut oil 1/3 cup pumpkin puree 1/3 cup almond oil
- ¼ cup almond oil
- ounces sugar-free dark chocolate
- 1 ½ teaspoon of pumpkin pie spice mix Stevia to taste

Directions:

2. Melt almond oil and dark chocolate over a double boiler. Take this mixture and layer the bottom of 12 muffin cups. Freeze until the crust has set. Meanwhile, take a saucepan and combine the rest of the ingredients.

3. Put the saucepan on low heat. Heat until softened and mix well. Pour this over the initial chocolate mixture. Let it chill within 1 hour, then serve.

Nutrition: Calories: 124 Carbs: 3g Fiber: 1g Protein: 3g Fat: 13g Sodium: 0mg

Sweet Almond and Coconut Fat Bomb

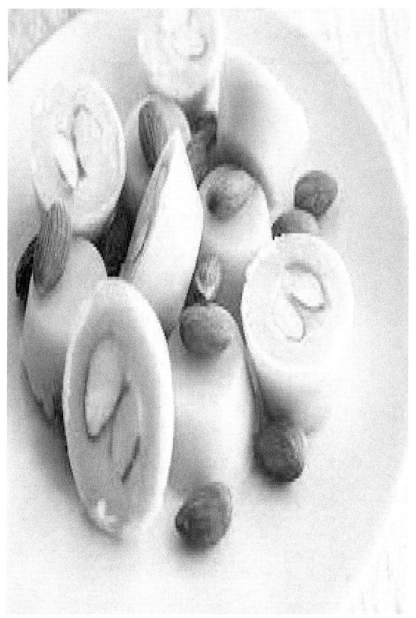

Preparation time:

10 minutes Cooking Time: 0 minutes Servings: 6

Ingredients:

- ¼ cup melted coconut oil
- 9 ½ tablespoons almond butter 90 drops liquid stevia
- 3 tablespoons cocoa
- 9 tablespoons melted butter, salted

Directions:

Take a bowl and add all of the listed ingredients. Mix them well. Pour scant 2 tablespoons of the mixture into as many muffin molds as you like. Chill for 20 minutes and pop them out. Serve and enjoy!

Nutrition: Calories: 72 Carbs: 2g Fiber: 0g Protein: 2.53g Fat: 14g Sodium: 0mg

Almond and Tomato Balls

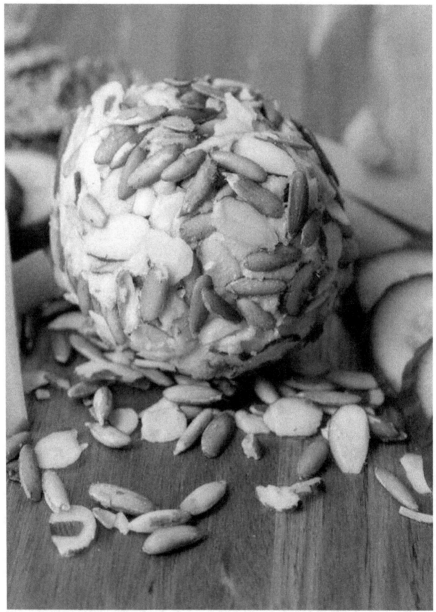

Preparation time:

10 minutes Cooking Time: 0 minutes Servings: 6

Ingredients:

- 1/3 cup pistachios, de-shelled 10 ounces cream cheese
- 1/3 cup sun-dried tomatoes, diced

Directions:

1. Chop pistachios into small pieces. Add cream cheese, tomatoes in a bowl and mix well. Chill for 15-20 minutes and turn into balls. Roll into pistachios. Serve and enjoy!

Nutrition: Calories: 183 Fat: 18g Carb: 5g Protein: 5g

Sodium: 10 mg

Avocado Tuna Bites

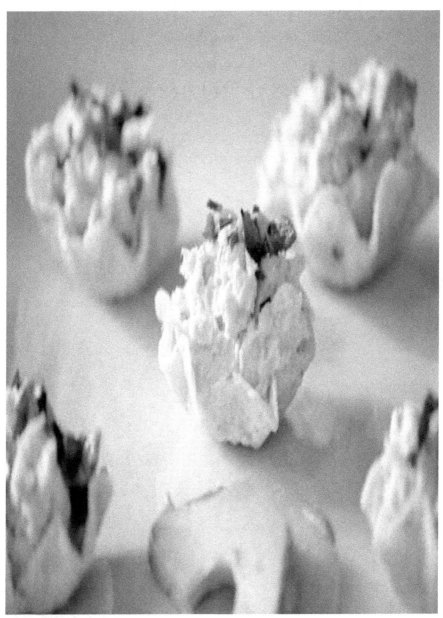

Preparation time:

10 minutes Cooking Time: 0 minutes Servings: 4

Ingredients:

- 1/3 cup coconut oil
- 1 avocado, cut into cubes
- 10 ounces of canned tuna, drained
- ¼ cup parmesan cheese, grated
- ¼ teaspoon garlic powder 1/4 teaspoon onion powder 1/3 cup almond flour
- ¼ teaspoon pepper
- ¼ cup low-fat mayonnaise Pepper as needed

Directions:

2. Take a bowl and add tuna, mayo, flour, parmesan, spices, and mix well. Fold in avocado and make 12 balls out of the mixture. Dissolve coconut oil in a pan and cook over medium heat until all sides are golden. Serve and enjoy!

Nutrition: Calories: 185 Fat: 18g

Carbohydrates: 1g Protein: 5g Sodium: 0mg

Faux Mac and Cheese

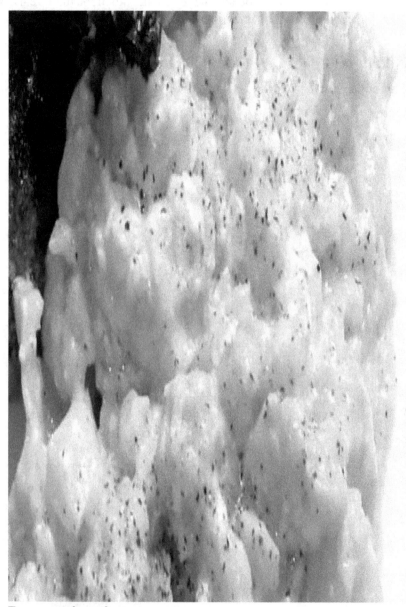

Preparation time:

15 minutes Cooking Time: 45 minutes Servings: 4

Ingredients:

- cups cauliflower florets Salt and pepper to taste
- cup of coconut milk
- ½ cup vegetable broth
- tablespoons coconut flour, sifted 1 organic egg, beaten
- 2 cups cheddar cheese

Directions:

1. Warm your oven to 350 degrees F. Season florets with salt and steam until firm. Place florets in a greased ovenproof dish. Heat-up coconut milk over medium heat in a skillet; make sure to season the oil with salt and pepper.

2. Stir in broth and add coconut flour to the mix, stir. Cook until the sauce begins to bubble. Remove heat and add beaten egg. Pour the thick sauce over cauliflower and mix in cheese. Bake for 30-45 minutes. Serve and enjoy!

Nutrition: Calories: 229 Fat: 14g

Carbohydrates: 9g Protein: 15g Sodium: 125 mg

Banana Custard

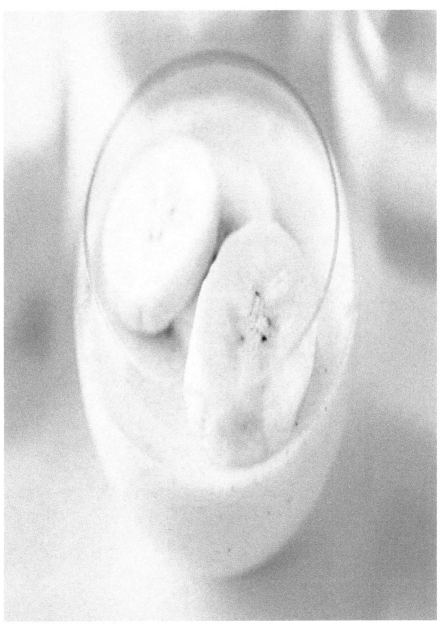

Preparation time:

10 minutes Cooking Time: 25 minutes Servings: 3

Ingredients:

- 2 ripe bananas, peeled and mashed finely
- ½ teaspoon of vanilla extract
- 14-onnce unsweetened almond milk 3 eggs

Directions:

1. Warm your oven to 350 degrees F. Grease 8 custard glasses lightly. Arrange the glasses in a large baking dish. Take a large bowl and mix all of the ingredients and mix them well until combined nicely.

2. Divide the mixture evenly between the glasses. Pour water into the baking dish. Bake for 25 minutes. Take out and serve.

Nutrition: Calories: 59 Fat: 2.4g

Carbohydrates: 7g Protein: 3g Sodium: 92 mg

Healthy Tahini Buns

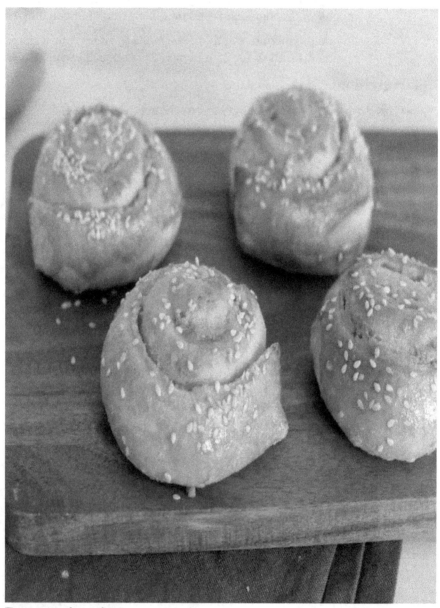

Preparation time:

10 minutes Cooking Time: 15-20 minutes Servings: 3

Ingredients:

- 1 whole egg
- 5 tablespoons Tahini paste
- ½ teaspoon baking soda 1 teaspoon lemon juice 1 pinch salt

Directions:

1. Warm your oven to 350 degrees F. Line a baking sheet with parchment paper and keep it on the side. Put the listed fixing in a blender and blend until you have a smooth batter.

2. Scoop batter onto prepared sheet forming buns. Bake for 15-20 minutes. Remove, then let them cool. Serve and enjoy!

Nutrition: Calories: 172 Carbs: 7g Fiber: 2g Protein: 6g Fat: 14g

Sodium: 112 mg

Chocolate Truffles

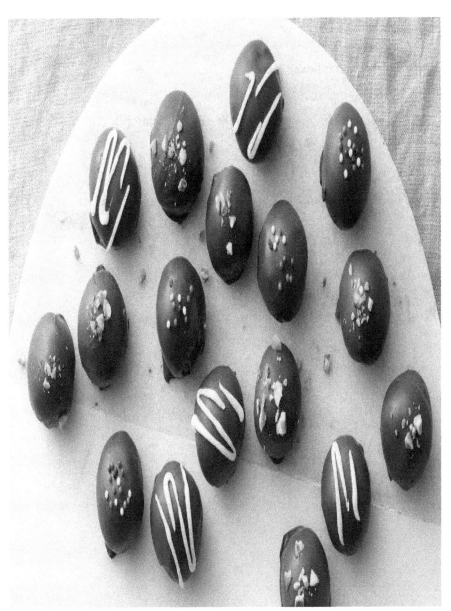

Preparation time:

15 minutes Cooking time: 0 minutes Servings: 24

Ingredients:

For the truffles:

- ½ cup cacao powder
- ¼ cup chia seeds
- ¼ cup flaxseed meal
- ¼ cup maple syrup 1 cup flour
- tablespoons almond milk For the Coatings:
- Cacao powder
- Chia seeds Flour
- Shredded coconut, unsweetened

Directions:

1. Place all the fixing for the truffle in a blender; pulse until it is thoroughly blended; transfer contents to a bowl. Form into chocolate balls, then cover with the coating ingredients. Serve immediately.

Nutrition: Calories 70

Sodium 2 mg

Fats 1 g

Carbohydrates 4 g

Fibers 2 g

Sugar 11 g

Proteins 1 g

Grilled Pineapple Strips

Preparation time:

15 minutes Cooking time: 5 minutes Servings: 6

Ingredients:

- Vegetable oil
- Dash of iodized salt 1 pineapple
- 1 tablespoon lime juice extract 1 tablespoon olive oil
- 1 tablespoon raw honey
- 3 tablespoons brown sugar

Directions:

1. Peel the pineapple, remove the eyes of the fruit, and discard the core.

2. Slice lengthwise, forming six wedges. Mix the rest of the fixing in a bowl until blended.

3. Brush the coating mixture on the pineapple (reserve some for basting). Grease an oven or outdoor grill rack with vegetable oil.

4. Place the pineapple wedges on the grill rack and heat for a few minutes per side until golden brownish, basting it frequently with a reserved glaze. Serve on a platter.

Nutrition: Calories 97

Fats 2 g

Carbohydrates 20 g

Sodium 2 mg

Sugar 17 g

Fibers 1 g

Proteins 1 g

Raspberry Peach Pancake

Preparation time:

15 minutes Cooking time: 30 minutes Servings: 4

Ingredients:

- ½ teaspoon sugar
- ½ cup raspberries
- ½ cup fat-free milk
- ½ cup all-purpose flour
- ¼ cup vanilla yogurt
- 1/8 teaspoon iodized salt 1 tablespoon butter
- 2 medium peeled, thinly sliced peaches 3 lightly beaten organic eggs

Directions:

1. Preheat oven to 400 °F. Toss peaches and raspberries with sugar in a bowl. Melt butter in a 9-inch round baking plate. Mix eggs, milk, plus salt in a small bowl until blended; whisk in the flour.

2. Remove the round baking plate from the oven, tilt to coat the bottom and sides with the melted butter; pour in the flour mixture.

3. Put it in the oven until it becomes brownish and puffed. Remove the pancake from the oven. Serve immediately with more raspberries and vanilla yogurt.

Nutrition: Calories 199

Sodium 173 mg

Fats 7 g

Cholesterol 149 g

Carbohydrates 25 g

Sugar 11 g

Fibers 3 g

Proteins 9 g

Mango Rice Pudding

Preparation time:

15 minutes Cooking time: 35 minutes Servings: 4

Ingredients:

- ½ teaspoon ground cinnamon
- ¼ teaspoon iodized salt
- 1 teaspoon vanilla extract
- cup long-grain uncooked brown rice 2 mediums ripe, peeled, cored mango 1 cup vanilla soymilk
- tablespoons sugar 2 cups of water

Directions:

1. Bring saltwater to a boil in a saucepan to cook rice; after a few minutes, simmer covered within 30-35 minutes until the rice absorbs the water. Mash the mango with a mortar and pestle or stainless-steel fork.

2. Pour milk, sugar, cinnamon, and the mashed mango into the rice; cook uncovered on low heat, stirring frequently. Remove the mango rice pudding from the heat, then stir in the vanilla soymilk. Serve immediately.

Nutrition: Calories 275

Sodium 176 mg

Fats 3 g

Carbohydrates 58 mg

Sugar 20 g

Fibers 3 g

Choco Banana Cake

Preparation time:

15 minutes Cooking time: 30 minutes Servings: 18

Ingredients:

- ½ cup semisweet dark chocolate
- ½ cup brown sugar
- ½ teaspoon baking soda
- ¼ cup unsweetened cocoa powder
- ¼ cup canola oil
- ¾ cup soymilk 1 large egg
- 1 egg white
- 1 large, ripe, mashed banana
- tablespoon lemon juice extract 1 teaspoon vanilla extract
- cups all-purpose flour

Directions:

1. Preheat the oven to 350 °F. Coat a baking pan with a non-stick spray. Whisk brown sugar, flour, baking soda, and cocoa powder in a bowl.

2. In another bowl, whisk bananas, lemon juice extract, vanilla extract, oil, soymilk, egg, and egg whites. Create a hole in the flour mixture's core or center, then pour in the banana mixture and mix in the dark chocolate.

3. Stir all the fixing with a spoon until thoroughly blended; spoon the batter onto the baking pan. Place in the oven and bake within 25-30 minutes until the center springs back when pressed lightly using your fingertips.

Nutrition:

Calories 150

Sodium 52 mg

Cholesterol 12 mg

Fats 3 g

Carbohydrates 27 g

Proteins 3 g

Zesty Zucchini Muffins

Preparation time:

15 minutes Cooking time: 30 minutes Servings: 12

Ingredients:

- Vegetable oil cooking spray
- ½ cup of sugar
- ¼ teaspoon iodized salt
- ¼ teaspoon ground nutmeg
- ¾ cup skim milk
- 1 cup shredded zucchini
- tablespoon baking powder 1 large egg
- teaspoons grated lemon rind
- 2 cups of all-purpose flour 3 tablespoons vegetable oil

Directions:

1. Mix the flour, baking powder, sugar, salt, plus lemon rinds in a bowl. Create a well in the center of the flour batter. In another bowl, mix zucchini, milk, vegetable oil, and egg. Coat muffin cups with vegetable oil cooking spray.

2. Divide the batter equally into 12 muffin cups. Transfer the muffin cups to the baking pan, put it in a microwave oven, and bake at 400 °F within 30 minutes until light golden brown. Remove, then allow to cool on a wire rack before serving.

Nutrition: Calories 169

Sodium 211.5 mg

Fats 4.8 g

Potassium 80.2 g

Carbohydrates 29.1 g

Fibers 2.5 g

Sugar 12.8 g

Proteins 0 g

Blueberry Oat Muffins

Preparation time:

15 minutes Cooking time: 30 minutes Servings: 12

Ingredients:

- ½ cup raw oatmeal
- ½ teaspoon baking powder
- ½ teaspoon iodized salt
- ½ cup dry milk
- ¼ cup of vegetable oil
- ¼ teaspoon baking soda 1/3 cup sugar
- 1 ½ cup flour 1 cup milk
- cup blueberries

Directions:

1. Preheat oven to 350 °F. Coat the muffin tins with vegetable oil. Mix or combine the flour, baking soda, baking powder, oats, sugar, and salt in a bowl. Mix milk, dry milk, egg, and vegetable oil in another bowl.

2. Pour the bowl of wet fixing into the bowl of dry fixing and mix partially. Add the blueberries and mix until the consistency turns lumpy. Scoop blueberry batter into the muffin tins.

3. Bake within 30 minutes until the muffins turn golden brown on the edges. Serve warm immediately or put it in an airtight container and store it in the refrigerator to chill.

Nutrition: Calories 150

Sodium 180 mg

Fats 5 g

Carbohydrates 22 g

Proteins 4 g

Fibers 1 g

Banana Bread

Preparation time:

15 minutes Cooking time: 60 minutes Servings: 14

Ingredients:

- Vegetable oil cooking spray
- ½ cup brown rice flour
- ½ cup amaranth flour
- ½ cup tapioca flour
- ½ cup millet flour
- ½ cup quinoa flour
- ½ cup of raw sugar
- ¾ cup egg whites
- 1/8 teaspoon iodized salt 1 teaspoon baking soda
- tablespoons grapeseed oil 2 pieces of mashed banana

Directions:

1. Preheat oven to 350 °F. Coat a loaf pan with a vegetable oil cooking spray, dust evenly with a bit of flour, and set aside. In a bowl, mix the brown rice flour, amaranth flour, tapioca flour, millet flour, quinoa flour, and baking soda

2. Coat a separate bowl with vegetable oil, then mix eggs, sugar, and mashed bananas. Pour the bowl of wet fixing into the bowl of dry fixing and mix thoroughly. Scoop the mixture into the loaf pan. Bake within an hour.

3. To check the doneness, insert a toothpick in the center of the loaf pan; if you remove the toothpick and it has no batter sticking to it, remove the bread from the oven. Slice and serve immediately and store the remaining banana bread in a refrigerator to prolong shelf life.

Nutrition: Calories 150

Sodium 150 mg

Fats 3 g

Fibers 2 g

Proteins 4 g

Sugar 7 g

Poached Pears

Preparation time:

15 minutes Cooking time: 30 minutes Servings: 4

Ingredients:

- ¼ cup apple juice extract
- ½ cup fresh raspberries
- cup of orange juice extract 1 teaspoon cinnamon, ground 1 teaspoon ground nutmeg
- tablespoons orange zest
- 4 whole pears, peeled, destemmed, core removed

Directions:

1. In a bowl, combine the fruit juices, nutmeg, and cinnamon, and then stir evenly. In a shallow pan, pour the fruit juice mixture, and set to medium fire.

2. Adjust the heat to simmer within 30 minutes; turn pears frequently to maintain poaching, do not boil. Transfer poached pears to a serving bowl; garnish with orange zest and raspberries.

Nutrition: Calories 140

Fats 0.5 g

Proteins 1 g

Carbohydrates 34 g

Fibers 2 g

Sodium 9 mg

Pumpkin with Chia Seeds Pudding

Preparation time:

60 minutes Cooking time: 0 minutes Servings: 4

Ingredients:

- For the Pudding:
- ½ cuporganic chia seeds
- ¼ cup raw maple syrup 1 ¼ cup low-fat milk
- cup pumpkin puree extract For the Toppings:
- ¼ cup organic sunflower seeds
- ¼ cup coarsely chopped almonds
- ¼ cup blueberries

Directions:

1. Add all the ingredients for the pudding in a bowl and mix until blended. Cover and store in a chiller for 1-hour. Remove from the chiller, transfer contents to a jar and add the ingredients for the toppings. Serve immediately.

Nutrition: Calories 189

Sodium 42 mg

Fats 7 g

Potassium 311 mg

Carbohydrates 27 g

Fibers 4 g

Proteins 5 g

Sugar 18 g

Milk Chocolate Pudding

Preparation time:

15 minutes Cooking time: 15 minutes Servings: 4

Ingredients:

- ½ teaspoon vanilla extract 1/3 cup chocolate chips 1/8 teaspoon salt
- 2 cups nonfat milk
- tablespoons cocoa powder 2 tablespoons sugar
- tablespoons cornstarch

Directions:

1. Mix cocoa powder, cornstarch, sugar, and salt in a saucepan and whisk in milk; frequently stir over medium heat.

2. Remove, put the chocolate chips and vanilla extract, stir until the chocolate chips and vanilla melt into the pudding. Pour contents into serving bowls and store in a chiller. Serve chilled.

Nutrition: Calories 197

Sodium 5 mg

Fats 5 g

Carbohydrates 9 g

Proteins 0.5 g

Minty Lime and Grapefruit Yogurt Parfait

Preparation time:

15 minutes Cooking time: 0 minutes Servings: 6

Ingredients:

- A handful of torn mint leaves 2 teaspoons grated lime zest
- tablespoons lime juice extract
- tablespoons raw honey 4 large red grapefruits
- cups reduced-fat plain yogurt

Directions:

1. Cut the top and lower part of the red grapefruits and stand the fruit upright on a cutting board. Discard the peel with a knife and slice along the membrane of each segment to remove the skin.

2. Mix yogurt, lime juice extract, and lime zest in a bowl. Layer half of the grapefruit and yogurt mixture into 6 parfait glasses; add another layer until the glass is filled and then drizzle with honey and top with mint leaves. Serve immediately.

Nutrition: Calories 207

Sodium 115 mg

Fats 3 g

Cholesterol 10 mg

Carbohydrates 39 mg

Sugar 36 g

Fibers 3 g

Peach Tarts

Preparation time:

15 minutes Cooking time: 55 minutes Servings: 8

Ingredients:

Tart Ingredients:

- ¼ cup softened butter
- ¼ teaspoon ground nutmeg 1 cup all-purpose flour
- 3 tablespoons sugar Filling **Ingredients:**
- ¼ teaspoon ground cinnamon
- ¼ cup coarsely chopped almonds 1/8 teaspoon almond extract
- 1/3 cup sugar
- 2 pounds peaches medium, peeled, thinly sliced

Directions:

1. Preheat oven to 375 °F. Mix butter, nutmeg, and sugar in a bowl until light and fluffy. Add and beat in flour until well-blended. Place the batter on an ungreased fluted tart baking pan and press firmly on the bottom and topsides.

2. Put it in the medium rack of the preheated oven and bake for about 10 minutes until it turns to a crust. In a bowl, coat peaches with sugar, flour, cinnamon, almond extract, and almonds.

3. Open the oven, put the tart crust on the lower rack of the oven, and pour in the peach filling; bake for about 40-45 minutes. Remove, cool, and serve; or cover with a cling wrap and refrigerate to serve chilled.

Nutrition: Calories 222

Sodium 46 milligrams

Fats 8 g

Cholesterol 15 mg

Carbohydrates 36 g

Sugar 21 g

Fibers 3 g

Proteins 4 g

Raspberry Nuts Parfait

Preparation time:

15 minutes Cooking time: 10 minutes Servings: 1

Ingredients:

- ¼ cup frozen raspberries
- ¼ cup frozen blueberries
- ¼ cup toasted, thinly sliced almonds 1 cup nonfat, plain Greek yogurt
- 2 teaspoons raw honey

Directions:

1. First, layer Greek yogurt in a parfait glass; add berries; layer yogurt again, top with almonds and more berries; drizzle with honey. Serve chilled.

Nutrition: Calories 378

Sodium 83 mg

Fats 15 g

Fibers 6 g

Carbohydrates 35 g

Proteins 30 g

Sugar 25 g

Strawberry Bruschetta

Preparation time:

15 minutes Cooking time: 0 minutes Servings: 12

Ingredients:

- 1 loaf sliced Ciabatta bread 8 ounces goat cheese
- cup basil leaves
- containers of strawberries, sliced 5 tablespoons balsamic glaze

Directions:

Wash and slice strawberries; set aside. Wash and chop the basil leaves; set aside. Slice the ciabatta bread and spread some goat cheese evenly on each slice; add strawberries, balsamic glaze, and top with basil leaves. Serve on a platter.

Nutrition: Calories 80

Sodium 59 mg

Fats 2 g

Carbohydrates 12 g

Proteins 3 g

Vanilla Cupcakes with Cinnamon-Fudge Frosting

Preparation time:

10 minutes Cooking Time: 18 minutes Servings: 1 dozen **Ingredients:**

- 11/2 cups white whole-wheat flour 3/4 cup sugar
- 3/4 teaspoon sodium-free baking powder
- 1/2 teaspoon sodium-free baking soda 1 cup nondairy milk
- 6 tablespoons canola oil
- tablespoon apple cider vinegar 1 tablespoon pure vanilla extract
- Frosting:
- cups powdered sugar
- 1/3 cup unsweetened cocoa powder
- 4 tablespoons non-hydrogenated vegetable shortening 4 tablespoons nondairy milk
- teaspoon ground cinnamon 1 teaspoon pure vanilla extract

Directions:

1. Warm oven to 350 F. Line a 12-muffin tin with paper liners and put aside. Mix or combine the flour, sugar, baking powder, and baking soda into a mixing bowl. Add the remaining batter fixing and stir just until combined.

2. Split the batter evenly between the muffin cups, then bake within 18 minutes. Remove, then put on a wire rack to cool. Beat until fluffy the frosting fixings into a mixing bowl. Frost cupcakes. Serve immediately.

Nutrition:

Calories: 347

Fat: 7 g

Protein: 13 g

Sodium: 46 mg

Fiber: 4 g

Carbohydrates: 60 g

Sugar: 3 g

Chocolate Cupcakes with Vanilla Frosting

Preparation time:

15 minutes Cooking time: 20 minutes Servings: 12

Ingredients:

- 11/2 cups white whole-wheat flour 1 cup of sugar
- teaspoons sodium-free baking soda
- 1/4 cup unsweetened cocoa powder 1 cup of water
- 4 tablespoons canola oil
- 4 tablespoons unsweetened applesauce 1 tablespoon pure vanilla extract
- 1 teaspoon distilled white vinegar
- Frosting:
- 11/2 cups powdered sugar
- 4 tablespoons non-hydrogenated vegetable shortening 21/2 tablespoons nondairy milk
- 1 tablespoon pure vanilla extract

Directions:

1. Warm oven to 350°F. Prepare a 12-muffin tin with paper liners and set aside. Measure the flour, sugar, and baking soda into a mixing bowl and whisk well to combine. Put the rest of the batter ingredients and stir just until combined.

2. Divide the batter evenly into the muffin cups. Bake within 20 minutes or until a toothpick inserted in the center of cupcakes comes out clean.

3. Remove, then put on a wire rack to cool. Mix the frosting fixing into a clean mixing bowl, then frost cupcakes. Serve immediately.

Nutrition:

Calories: 272

Fat: 9 g

Protein: 2 g

Sodium: 2 mg

Fiber: 1 g

Carbohydrates: 45 g

Sugar: 32 g

Alphabetical Index